Learning How To Eat (Again)

by Brian V. Menard

This Book Is Dedicated to the memory
of my best friend and cherished wife.
"Heaven must have been short an Angel."
Elsie L. Menard
1950 - 1997

AUTHOR'S COMMENT

If something is not broken, then why fix it? This cliché reflects the attitudes of many people worldwide. But, when it comes to taking responsibility for our health, should this attitude still apply? Unfortunately, this was the attitude I used to have regarding my weight problem. My blood pressure was fine, I had a hearty appetite and I felt great. Besides, losing weight is a real drag. First you starve yourself, then you have to buy new clothes and then you gain all the weight right back again (usually with a few pounds of interest). Dieting was certainly not my idea of a "good time". There has got to be a better way! So then, what are the alternatives? Diet pills, powdered diet drinks, prepackaged diet meals, frequent "fasting", abnormal amounts of exercise, "Fad" diets, Lypo-suction, surgical stomach shrinking or "rabbit food"?! NO THANK YOU! I'll pass on all of these options! But what is the alternative? Obesity?

Fortunately, there is a solution. But before you can implement a solution, you must first understand the problem. The problem is fat; not calories, not cholesterol, not sugar but fat! Not saturated fat, not polyunsaturated fat, and not even monounsaturated fat but "*all fats.*" Fat, the whole fat and nothing but the fat. All of these other items may have problems unto themselves but when it comes down to weight control, FAT steals the show! Until you learn to fully master the art of controlling your daily fat intake (DFI) you will never be able to claim total victory over your appetite! Learning to master your daily fat intake or "DFI" is really not that difficult but it does require a deliberate effort and a discerning eye. With practice, though, anyone can do it. In the following pages, I will explain in detail how to gain control of your DFI quickly and easily. You may never look at weight control the same ever again.

CHAPTERS

OUTLINE

INTRODUCTION

    A. Basic introduction
    B. My reason for writing this book

I............DEFINING THE PROBLEM

    A. Eating problem in America
        1.Eating the wrong foods
        2.Confusion regarding proper nutrition
    B. A pattern developed
        1.Eating less meat
        2.More rich food
        3.Compensation for lost fat

II...........WHAT ABOUT FAT?

    A .Searching for healthful foods
    B The real enemy
    C Labeling of food products
        1.The need to read all labels
        2 Monitoring daily fat intake (DFI)
        3.Honesty in labeling
    D. Eating totally "fat free"
        1.Why initial attempts failed
        2.Acceptable allowances of fat
        3.The ease of eating high fat
    E. Generally accepted guidelines aren't sufficient

III.........DAILY FAT INTAKE (DFI)

        A. Determining fat content
        B. Illustrating the need for examining
           all foods
        C. Description of some high fat foods
           1.Reducing fat intake gradually
           2.The need to eat sufficient quantity
        D. Simple changes which yield great results
        E. Benefits of eating less fat
           1. Weight loss
           2. Better health
           3. Lower cholesterol levels
           4. Less expensive
           5.More energy

IV.........AN UNAWARE PUBLIC

        A. Eating high fat foods unconsciously
        B. Converting healthy food to unhealthy food
        C. The effect of limiting fat by the grams
        D. Healthier foods follow naturally
        E.Products without nutritional information labels

V.........TWENTY SPECIAL COINS

        A. Purpose of coins
        B. Where and when to invest
        C. Some favorite recipes
        D. Avoid getting too hungry.

VI.........TEN EASY CHANGES

        Ten ways to reduce your daily fat intake (DFI)
        without missing it.

VII........OH NUTS!

    A. Eating nuts on a low-fat diet
    B. Steak vs. nuts
    C. Avoid as a snack
    D. Other foods requiring moderation
        1. Olives
        2. Cheese(s)
        3. Beverages

VIII........OBSERVATIONS ON LOSING WEIGHT

    A. The need for an accurate scale
    B. Testing your scale for accuracy
    C. Eating to "please the scale"
    D. Observation # 1
        1. On weight loss while sleeping
        2. On drinking enough fluids
    E. Observation # 2
        1. Weight loss fluctuations
        2. The need to avoid "eating to please your scale"
    F. Observation # 3
        1. Good nutrition as a habit
        2. Skipping meals
        3. Cultivating good eating habits

IX..........SNACKING

    A. To be done only as a dessert
    B. Ultimately causes poor nutrition
    C. Overweight people are not "over-nourished"
    D. Beware of "Diet sodas"

X...........MAINTENANCE AND SETTING GOALS

      A. Reintroducing foods into your diet
      B. Setting realistic goals
         1. Start with long term goals
         2. Understand your body's needs before setting short term goals

XI..........WATER

      A. The need to drink more
      B. Free use of

XII.........CHEATING OR "DAYS OFF"

      A. Making provisions for
      B. The need to still observe meal times
      C. Cheating all day
      D. Using "Days off" for eating out

XIII.........EATING OUT

      A. Reasons for eating out
         1. As opposed to skipping meals
         2. Sometimes cannot be avoided
      B. Reasons we should not "eat out"
         1. To reward our success
         2. Convenience
         3. Difficult to monitor DFI
         4. Usually very high fat contents
      C. Suggestions for "eating out"

LEARNING HOW TO EAT (AGAIN)

INTRODUCTION

With all the concern about health and fitness these days, thousands of food and clothing manufacturers have rushed to our rescue with everything from thermonuclear tennis shoes to non-fat cheesecake! We seem to live in a world full of extremes. There has recently been a lot of publicity about eating a "low-fat" diet (along with many other popular suggestions). Unfortunately, much of this advice overwhelms us.

We are advised to monitor our fat consumption by eating foods that are at least 70 – 80% fat free. Opinions may vary on these percentages but these are the most commonly advised allowances. This method may work quite effectively at first but soon you find yourself gaining the weight back that you so diligently labored to lose. The problem is that eating on this type of program, you have to carefully monitor calories as well as fat percentages and maybe even the actual types of fat (saturated and unsaturated). If you are not careful, you could find yourself in worse shape than you were when you started out. So what is a person to do?

Fortunately there is an easy solution. In this book, I will explain the methods that allowed me to lose over 50 pounds in only seven months without ever needing to go hungry! In addition, I can now maintain my weight with ease. Losing (or gaining) weight is no longer a problem.

I NOW HAVE TOTAL CONTROL OF MY WEIGHT!

Have you ever wanted to say this? Until recently, it seemed like this was a matter of luck or perhaps even fate to be fat or thin. However, it doesn't require any luck at all. There are several things you must understand, but you can control your weight. If I can do it, I'm certain that anyone can do it. I am certainly no pillar of self control and even I managed to regain total control in only three months!

That's right, total control! After an entire lifetime of struggling to control my weight, Victory is finally mine! It can be yours also if you want it to be! Everything you need to know about controlling your weight is contained in the following pages.

(1)

DEFINING THE PROBLEM

Americans have a serious eating problem. We are obsessed with high fat foods. Several factors have contributed to this dilemma. Fast food restaurants, Television advertising, and a society that is generally Hedonistic by nature have all played a major role in the degeneration of our appetites. In addition, it seems as though prepackaged food manufacturers have sold our nutritional needs down the proverbial river. We are deceived into "so-called" healthy breakfasts of doughnuts and toaster pastries, healthy "French Fries" and "Deluxe" cheeseburgers for lunch and home delivered pizza for a "nutritious" supper. Who is kidding who here?! There are countless numbers of healthy products on the market if you can just figure out which ones. The problem is that with both healthy and unhealthy products being labeled as good for you, it has become somewhat of a shell game to find <u>real nutrition</u>!

In my initial quest for good nutrition, I often found myself on the verge of a nervous breakdown while trying to locate foods that were low in fat, calories, salt, cholesterol, MSG, preservatives, artificial colors and so on... It was beginning to appear that some of the healthiest products weren't in the packages, but were the packages themselves. I was quickly becoming disenchanted. There had to be an easier way. Learning to eat sensibly in an insensible world is challenging at best but the good news is... it is possible. If I can do it, anyone can do it!

WHAT ABOUT FAT?

How many times have you seen a person in a grocery store studying the label on an item off the shelf? Probably quite often, right? It seems as if everyone is looking for something (or perhaps the lack of something), for various health-related reasons. Some may be looking for sodium, while others perhaps cholesterol, others still may be monitoring calories and sugar. What are all these people really looking for? Do they check every single item? Are they all totally paranoid? Well, perhaps any of these suggestions could apply to some of the people on occasion but I suspect that most people checking nutritional labels are usually targeting only one or two specific items. People with high blood pressure are probably more concerned with salt and cholesterol, "dieters" with calories and sugar. Yet, the real enemy in the pantry will often slip by us undetected. You guessed it … FAT!

It is not my intention to discredit the shortfalls of other problem items, but fat is the overweight person's worst enemy and most people don't even realize it! Until you become aware of the fat content in every single item you eat, you will never have total control of your appetite or your weight! You see, fat defies calorie monitoring. It breaks all the traditional rules about calories' relationship to weight gain in our bodies. Therefore, if you learn how to control your daily fat intake (DFI), you will no longer need to worry about counting calories. This is why it is so important to read every label on every single item until you are totally aware of the many places fat is hidden! This may seem fanatical, but until you become familiar with the foods that you regularly eat, or intend to start eating as part of a new fat-watch program, this is absolutely the most important step you can take towards modifying your daily fat intake (DFI).

As you do this, you will probably be amazed at how much fat is contained in foods never before suspected.

We are in desperate need of honest labeling on packaged foods in this country. When I first began watching fat contents, I felt as though I would starve to death the first few weeks. Most of the foods promoting "good health" were loaded with fat. I really didn't know how much fat I should have been eating but I was trying to keep my diet as fat-free as possible at first just to establish what level of fat would become most desirable. I quickly learned that it is simply not possible to eat totally fat-free. Even some fruits and vegetables contain small amounts of fat. Therefore, if fat-free is not possible, what then, is the lowest possible amount of fat you can consume and still eat like a normal person (as opposed to a rabbit)? I soon learned that if you are very careful, eventually it is relatively easy to stay below 20 grams per day and function at a normal or above normal level. I personally experience considerably more energy when I eat only 20 grams of fat per day.

However, you can exceed this number faster than you can say "cheesecake", if you don't take care to monitor your fat intake very closely. When I first started eating low-fat, I was surprised to learn that almost every single product I was typically eating was extremely high in fat. I had suspected that many items I had been eating could have been a little high in fat but because I ate only once or twice a day, I thought it really didn't matter. Back then I would often eat two or three snacks during the course of the day, in place of breakfast or lunch and then eat a large supper. Little did I realize that there was more fat in those couple of snacks alone than I needed for the entire day. Supper was often more than ten times the amount of fat that I now consume in a typical day. On the days that I ate out, I would sometimes do even worse, and I ate out quite often.

The American Heart Association has published a book called "Fat and Cholesterol Counter". In this book I found a formula for determining the maximum amount of calories that I should consume daily as well as the maximum amount of saturated and unsaturated fats that should be consumed. From these guidelines, I determined that if I were eating to maintain my ideal weight, I should consume no more than 88grams of fat per day and that no more than 26 of these should be from saturated fats. It is important to realize that these are only approximate maximum numbers. Approximate because everyone's activity levels and metabolic rates differ and maximum because, just like our speed limits, it is perfectly acceptable and perhaps even desirable to stay below the limit. Usually a little below the limit is the ideal.

In the case of fat consumption, how much below is the optimal amount? Is there such a thing as too low? How do we determine where to draw the line? One thing is certain, following any of the generally accepted guidelines you will never need to concern yourself with weight loss. This is because you will not be losing any weight! However, using the information for maximum amounts to consume, I proceeded to personally research the cause and effect of fat on weight control with some remarkable discoveries.

DAILY FAT INTAKE

When I first began monitoring my DFI (daily fat intake), it seemed almost impossible to determine the total grams of fat unless I wrote down each and every item of food and then carefully analyzed the content in each one. For example, a turkey sandwich made with low fat turkey breast slices may appear to be low fat. If properly prepared, it may be very low indeed. Unfortunately, when prepared in a traditional manner, any significant benefit from using low-fat turkey is lost. See example:

Example:

TYPICAL TURKEY SANDWICH

1 - 1 oz. slice turkey breast..............................2 grams fat

2 - slices whole wheat bread........................4 grams fat

1 - tablespoon of mayonnaise.......................10 grams fat

1 - 1 oz. slice American cheese......................9 grams fat

1 - tablespoon of butter (on bread)...............12 grams fat

Total..............37 grams fat x 2 (sandwiches) = **74 grams fat**

As you can see, my seemingly innocent and apparently low fat sandwiches have suddenly turned into a meal fit for "Jabba the Hut"! Believe It or not, each of these sandwiches is higher in fat than a quarter-pound cheeseburger at the local fast food restaurant!

Below is a brief sample of the foods I used to typically eat during the course of the week.

Cheeseburgers	Fast food sandwiches
French fries	Potato chips
Pizza	Cheesecake
Gourmet Ice Cream	Spaghetti and meatballs
Noodles Alfredo	Peanut butter cups
Candy bars	Whole Milk
Regular salad dressings	Cheese(s)
Snack crackers	Microwave popcorn
Cold cuts	Steak
Eggs	Prepackaged entrees
Burritos	Cookies
Brownies	Macaroni and cheese
Chili	Lasagna

I think it would be realistic to say that a week would rarely pass without having eaten most of the foods on this list at least one or more times. At this point, if you are seeing any serious parallels between my list and the foods you typically eat, you may be seriously contemplating burning this book! Please don't! I am not suggesting that you give up these foods, or any other favorite foods you might have. I am only saying that we need to read the fat content of all the foods we usually buy until we are so familiar with their content, we can determine the approximate quantity without seeing a label. This can only be done if you use the same foods regularly.

Until you have determined your own personal need for fat in your diet, you should experiment with the amount that you are personally consuming and reduce the amount at a rate no greater than 20% per week. Your body will immediately notice the fat reduction and if you reduce the intake too dramatically, you will feel hungry all the time. Please be careful to avoid letting yourself go hungry due to deprivation. This will almost certainly end in failure. Always allow yourself plenty of nutritious low-fat foods at every meal. If you do this and ration only the fat, you will find that you feel less groggy after meals and will experience more energy as well. Remember that turkey sandwich mentioned earlier? Now consider it's low-fat counterpart:

LOW-FAT TURKEY SANDWICH

1- 1oz slice low-fat turkey breast……..................…..2 grams fat

2- slices whole wheat bread (2 grams ea.)...........…4 grams fat

1- tablespoon of fat-free mayonnaise……............…0 grams fat

¼" thick tomato slice…........…….……...……...0 grams fat

2 oz. serving of crisp lettuce...........……...…........0 grams fat

Total................6 grams fat x 2 (sandwiches) = **12 grams fat**

As you can see, by changing a few simple ingredients, it is easy to reduce the total fat of these two sandwiches by 62 grams without even using low-fat bread. You also get to use the same sandwich meat. In fact you could even double the amount of sandwich meat and still be low in fat. In the low fat sandwich example you may want to note that I used a non-fat mayonnaise to spread on the bread in place of butter or margarine. This works quite well. Although 62 grams of fat may seem insignificant, consider this – most adults need less than 62 grams of fat for the entire day and many adults would exceed their maximum recommended allowance for fat with with this same amount.

I am six-foot-three and I have discovered that I feel best when limiting my fat intake to only 20 grams per day. I eat just as much food now as I did when I was overweight, only now I have found myself eating much healthier. I had reached a point before when I had actually lost my taste for fruits and vegetables. Breads and cereals held little appeal as well. These same foods now constitute a major portion of my daily intake. One of the wonderful benefits of reducing your daily fat intake is weight loss. Basically, it is very difficult to gain weight without consuming a considerable amount of fat daily. Thus, if you dramatically reduce your DFI, you will easily lose weight (unless you are already at your ideal weight).

While eating 20 grams of fat daily, based on a weekly average, I would typically lose from 1 – 3 pounds each day at first. Later the average loss settled to a very respectable ½ - 1 pound per day. The thing is, I kept on losing at this rate as long as I maintained only 20 grams of fat per day. It almost seems strange to eat so well and still lose weight. It didn't hurt that I felt great doing it, also. However, weight loss is not the only benefit experienced while eating "ultra low-fat" on this plan, you can also expect to feel better, dramatically decrease your cholesterol intake level and have more energy as well! This is why I had to write this book – to let you know that it is possible to learn how to eat properly without going to special prepackaged meals or paying for costly clinics. A greater awareness of your DFI is the secret to easy weight control.

AN UNAWARE PUBLIC

Little things mean a lot!

Most of the people I have spoken to thus far concerning DFI (daily fat intake), seem to already be aware that they need to be monitoring their fat intake. However, (like myself at first), they don't seem to realize that large amounts of fat can show up where you least expect it. I am convinced that this is one of the major reasons that most of us fail at dieting.

We can easily point our finger in the denouncing of a banana split but when it comes to recognizing fat in such typical foods as toast, milk, sandwiches and small snacks, we are usually totally unaware of their contents. Now, don't get me wrong, I am not trying to suggest that you should avoid these foods, I am simply stating that these are some of the foods which we don't concern ourselves with when perhaps we should. In many cases I believe that we consume most of our fat intake unknowingly. We sometimes limit our intake of the obviously rich foods but we rarely concern ourselves with basic condiments. This is a huge oversight. In many instances, the condiments constitute the major fat content of a meal. This is sometimes true even when the meal is high in fat to begin with!

Consider a typical American breakfast. The following page begins with a list of just a few typical foods most of us have enjoyed at some time.

Eggs – Pancakes – Waffles – Toast – Muffins – Croissants –

Bagels – Doughnuts – Coffee cake – English muffins –

Cereals - Rolls and breads.

Although many of these foods are sometimes low in fat (and in some instances, even fat-free), every one of these items has the potential to be high in fat depending upon the way it is served and the initial ingredients.

In addition, many diligent shoppers will buy low-fat products only to later convert them back to a state worse than the original. Case in point: I have seen people fry cholesterol free and fat-free eggs at home in real butter or margarine and then serve along with a couple of slices of buttered toast. Granted this is hardly the crime of the century, but it is self defeating. If they had known how to prepare the food properly, it would have been very low in fat.

However, because they didn't know any better, most of the benefit was lost. Few people realize that there is more fat in a tablespoon of butter or margarine than you would typically find in two large fried eggs! If you then consider that toast can often require a full tablespoon of butter (or margarine) for each slice, it quickly becomes apparent that there is a serious need to closely monitor these items. The point here is not to condemn any particular food or the person preparing it, but rather to bring awareness to a much higher level than it is presently.

We can still enjoy any foods we previously enjoyed, the only difference is, now we can determine cause and effect. This knowledge is essential if we wish to control our weight. If I, for example, should decide that I would like to reduce my current weight by ten pounds, I know that I can achieve this goal in three weeks if I consume less than 20 grams of total fat per day during this period. No additional physical activity is necessary. Diet aids, special foods in frozen packages and appetite-controlling drugs are not necessary either.

Now, if I choose to do this, I know that I will have to plan my meals carefully and that many foods simply will not be consumed freely during this three week period. Some of the foods that will be monitored carefully are French Fries, pizza, grilled burgers and gourmet ice cream. There is simply no way you can eat these kinds of foods freely and stay under 20 grams of total fat for the day. I will, however, be eating a lot of fruits and vegetables. I have found that fruits and vegetables can be very satisfying when accompanied by hearty whole grain breads and rolls. Sandwiches made with fat-free mayonnaise, mustard or sandwich dressings can sometimes make you forget that you are eating on a low-fat budget. Many of the sandwich meats currently available are only one or two grams of fat per slice, thus allowing you the freedom to enjoy two or three of these sandwiches per day with little negative consequences.

While monitoring my fat intake during this period, I will not purchase any products that I intend to eat unless it has a nutritional information section on the label. I have found that if it isn't listed, it's usually because they figured that you really don't want to know just how unhealthy it is. During these three weeks, I will also make it a point to carefully examine each item being used in every meal. This may sound tedious but eventually you get used to recognizing what is and is not allowable and the approximate fat content in each item you typically eat.

When you reach this point (usually after two or three months), you will then discover that controlling your DFI becomes very easy.

TWENTY SPECIAL COINS

What exactly is a gram of fat? We hear this terminology quite frequently but do we really know what it means? For many of us, probably not. However, we are not to blame for our ignorance. We have received a great deal of help from the commercial food packaging industry. Allow me to illustrate; imagine driving into a local service station to purchase some gasoline. The price on the pump, that you have chosen to use, is listed at $3.75 per gallon. You then proceed to fill your tank. However, something strange begins to happen. You notice that as you fill your gas tank, the quantity display is showing you that you have just pumped over sixty pounds of gasoline into your car. How long would you continue to patronize that service station?

What possible motive could there be for charging you by the gallon but monitoring by the pound? Actually, there is a logical answer why certain gas stations might do this. If it happens to be an airport gas station, many pilots need to be concerned with the "pounds" of fuel they have in their planes.

But what does this have to do with grams and food? It's really quite simple. We wouldn't tolerate a gas station pulling such a stunt, yet we tolerate this exact same scenario from the prepared food industry. A gram is nothing more than a metric unit of weight measure, one one-thousandth of a kilogram. Simple enough right? So why are we given the quantities of our food by the pound or ounce and the ingredients by the metric system? If I told you that there was 28 grams of fat in your cheeseburger, would you know what I was talking about? If instead I told you that there was a full ounce of pure fat in that cheeseburger, would that make any more sense? How about if I were to tell you that many Americans consume over 200 grams of fat per day. Would that mean much to you? Well, how about if I told you that many Americans eat about 8 ounces of pure fat each day. Would that make more sense? If you learned that new research has indicated that most Americans should consume less than 60 grams of fat per day, would you know how to monitor your intake properly? Isn't it time we say enough is enough?

We are all far too intelligent to be deceived by these silly attempts by food manufactures. Lets beat them at their own game. How you ask? It's quite simple. Monitor our daily fat intake on our own terms. This is quite easy to do. All you need to do is limit the total number of grams of fat you allow yourself to consume daily. If you do this diligently, you will avoid their silly attempts to deceive you. There are many ways that this can be accomplished.

One of the methods I use to monitor my daily fat intake is to imagine having 20 special coins. Each one of these coins can be used for only one purpose; to purchase a gram of fat. I then consider that I can eat anything I desire but I can buy only 20 grams worth of fat. All other foods are free. So now the question is…do I want to spend all 20 grams on that cheeseburger, knowing that I will then need to eat "fat free" the rest of the day? Or would I perhaps care to invest a few grams here and a few grams there? I usually will visualize myself as an investor, typically investing in a few grams for breakfast, perhaps 12 grams at lunch, and the balance on supper or a snack. This is actually fun once you learn how to do it. Especially once you learn which foods will satisfy you that have little or no fat. One of the discoveries I have made is that fat tends to make the appetite rage out of control if eaten in highly concentrated forms.

For this reason, I tend to steer away from snacks during the day. I can inhale enough fat for the week in just a few moments if I permit myself to indulge in potato chips, cookies and candy bars (all of which are extremely high in fat). However, the inverse of this statement is also true. The less fat is consumed, the easier it is to control your appetite. Herein lies the secret to easy weight control!

A couple of times earlier, I referred to certain rules that must be followed. Of these rules, perhaps the most important, is to NEVER let yourself get overly hungry. Now, I'm not talking about working up a healthy appetite. No, not by any means. What I'm saying is, with this new-found control, you may find it is very easy to skip meals. I have found this to be disastrous on every occasion that I allowed it to happen. If you allow yourself to get overly hungry, the body seems to call out for more food than you need, and once this happens, I have found that the appetite will always have its way. It is better to over-eat at a meal than to allow yourself to get into this scenario.

(6)

TEN CHANGES TO CONSIDER

Another important rule is to never use butter or margarine freely! This, in my opinion, is the most overlooked source of high fat. Typically, a tablespoon of butter or margarine will range from 10 to 14 grams. When you consider that it is easy to use a full tablespoon on a single slice of toast or half of an English muffin, you can see how easy it would be to exceed your 20 gram allowance before you even begin eating your morning bowl of cereal! I know of several nice restaurants that consider a full order of toast to be four slices. At this rate, you could be getting as much as 52 grams of fat (including bread) before you even get started on their big breakfast special. If you happen to have opted for the slam bam breakfast special with hash browns, three eggs, toast, juice, breakfast meat and coffee with half and half, you could easily be looking down the barrel of a whopping 125 grams of fat. Wow! That really is a Slam Bam breakfast, isn't it!

I'm not suggesting that you never eat out; I'm only saying that you need to be aware that watching your fat consumption at a restaurant takes a very discerning eye. If you don't consider every item carefully, you will certainly go way over any reasonable amount of DFI. This is true of almost all restaurants! On a brighter note, by making a few relatively simple adjustments in your home, you can drastically reduce your DFI and not even miss the fat!

On the following pages, I'll show some easy examples to consider which will dramatically decrease your daily fat intake. Although these changes may seem insignificant, they can reduce you DFI dramatically. Sometimes by as much as

50%. If you can implement the ideas below into your daily routine, you will be half way there!

1). *Buy only 1% low-fat milk (or skim milk).*

One percent low-fat milk has less than half of the fat content found in two-percent low-fat milk.

e.g. –   8oz. 1% low-fat milk = 2 grams of fat
            8oz. 2% low-fat milk = 5 grams of fat

Skim milk has even less fat but, to me, the sacrifice is not worth it. It doesn't taste as good. And as you can see, drinking the 1% low-fat milk, you can easily have a bowl of cereal for breakfast with little consequence. Whereas using the 2% low-fat milk, your bowl of cereal would have to be considered the main meal of the day. I refuse to pay 5 special coins just for my cereal! However, 2 grams of fat will suit my daily budget quite nicely.

2). *Try switching to a "reduced fat" margarine.*

I use the term "reduced fat" deliberately because in my honest opinion, there is not as yet, any real low-fat variety available. At least, none with a melting point that will allow it to melt on toast and cooked vegetables. The brands presently available will typically be in the 6-8 grams per tablespoon range. Although this is certainly an improvement over the regular brands of margarine, it still warrants judicious application.

3). *Consider using "Fat free" ice cream and frozen yogurts.*

If you like ice cream, switch to a fat-free variety or a no-fat frozen yogurt. Once again, you will find it necessary to check all labels because not all frozen yogurts are fat-free. This adjustment need not be a hardship, though; there are several excellent varieties of low-fat and no-fat yogurts as well as ice cream choices presently available. Sampling different ones regularly is a burden that I will often place upon myself. It's a tough job, but somebody has to do it!

4). *Switch to very "low-fat" or "no-fat" salad dressing.*

I have noticed that some of these new salad dressings taste so good, it would be difficult to discern them from the regular version in a taste test.

5). *Reasons to use "fat-free" mayonnaise.*

Mayonnaise is one of those foods that actually seem to benefit from having the fat removed. It tastes better to me than the regular versions. It would appear that the reason for this is because the primary contributors to the fat content are the egg yolks and the oil. They do not seem to affect the taste very much but they add about 10 grams of fat per tablespoon to the mayonnaise. To be totally honest, I never really liked mayonnaise very much before I discovered the fat-free version. Also, please be aware of mayonnaise(s) that only claim to be "lite" or "low-fat" but, in fact, still contain almost as much fat as the regular varieties. One of the great side benefits of fat-free mayonnaise is that it can be used in place of the butter on your sandwich's bread and you'll hardly notice the difference! By switching to "no-fat" mayonnaise in your sandwiches it is easy to reduce your DFI by as much as 100 grams without even noticing the loss. Below is a comparison of a typical tuna sandwich with its low-fat counterpart on the next page.

Regular Tuna Sandwich:
1-Bulkie roll…………………….....................…....…..2 grams
3 oz. tuna w/ mayonnaise…….…...…............….............32 grams
1 oz. slice cheese………………….....…..............……9 grams
1 tbsp. Margarine……………………….......…..……..10 grams
Total grams per sandwich……....................…..….53 grams

Now Consider the "low-fat" alternative...

Low Fat Tuna Sandwich:

Bulkie roll…………………….......................…......…..2 grams
Tuna in water (3 oz.)……….........…......................….....1 gram
4 oz. fat-free mayonnaise…….……...............…........….0 grams
1 - slice of tomato………...…...........…..............…..…0 grams
2oz. crisp lettuce ……..........................….................…..0 grams
1 slice (1 oz.) low-fat cheese…...……….............…......2 grams
Total grams per sandwich……....................................5 grams

*Note: These items reflect fat contents in brands that I presently use. Low-fat foods can vary dramatically in their fat content. Please be sure to check each label carefully.

As you can see, the low-fat sandwich contains less than one-tenth as much fat as its traditional counterpart yet I can assure you that you will not miss the fat. Incidentally, you can do this with chicken or turkey salad sandwiches as well.

The illustrations I present from time to time are not intended to be a dietary guideline but are given only to demonstrate how easily fat can be reduced from a meal.

When the study of my personal eating habits first began, I calculated that my daily consumption was approximately 220 grams of fat per day. As time went on, I realized that this figure was actually an understatement. There had been several foods I had not made any allowances for. In addition, my calculations were extremely inaccurate for the fat contents being consumed when visiting restaurants. Unfortunately, most restaurants do not give nutritional information on their menus, therefore, I will perhaps never truly know exactly how much fat I was regularly consuming.

However, looking back now and recalculating, I would have to increase my initial estimate to be more realistic at 240-300 grams per day! Eating this much fat was easier to do than one might imagine. One of the reasons I regularly consumed so much fat was because I frequently ate at fast food stores and restaurants. It is easy for a guy my size to blow away 100 grams of fat in one meal and not even know he was doing anything wrong. Although I could cite several other good reasons for cooking at home, this is probably one of the best. If you choose to cook more at home, step #6 is absolutely essential.

6). Purchase a high quality, non-stick surface frying pan (unless you are already using one).

If you are going to take this new style of eating seriously, you owe it to yourself to invest in your health and use a good quality, non-stick pan. With some of the better models, you can cook with dramatically reduced amounts of cooking oil, margarine, butter or fat. And in some cases, you can actually fry with no fats or oils at all! While using these pans, you will find that you can enjoy just a touch of oil or butter for the taste, and still consume very little fat.

Recently, I developed a recipe for non-fat pancakes which are prepared without any fat or oil in a non-stick frying pan. There are several very desirable toppings which can be used (in addition to syrup) that will make you feel like you are having a gourmet breakfast and still be non-fat.

e.g. warm fruit compote, sprinkled confectioners' sugar, canned fruit such as crushed pineapple, or just use your imagination and create some of your own. One of my favorite ways to start the day is to finish a great tasting breakfast and walk away from the table with all 20 of my special coins still in my pocket to spend later. Perhaps for a couple of great sandwiches, which brings us to…

7). Cold cuts and sandwich meats...

Here again, you may find yourself actually preferring the low-fat versions to the original. Typically, a regular slice of sandwich meat (1 oz.) will contain about 8-10 grams of fat. The low-fat versions will generally have only about one or two grams of fat. I am not certain why, but bologna seems to always be a little bit higher. You will rarely see low-fat versions of bologna.

8). Fresh meats and poultry...

Try using meat as you would use a seasoning. While these items may be consumed within the guidelines of your new eating style, extreme caution is advised! It is very easy to consume several times your daily allotment for fat accidentally if you are not familiar with the contents of fresh meats and poultry and still consume them regularly. If you intend to eat meat regularly, it is highly advisable that you should obtain a fat counter book of some kind. I would personally recommend the "<u>American Heart Association's Fat and Cholesterol Counter</u>" booklet. It's a pocket size reference guide with a wealth of very useful information.

9). Fruits and Vegetables...

You should always strive to keep plenty of fruits and vegetables available to yourself at all times. Although fresh foods are generally preferred, canned, dried, and frozen are great alternatives. The amount of fat contained in fruits and vegetables is so low; I don't even bother calculating an allowance for it. I allow myself all that I want. By supplementing regular meals with plenty of fruits and vegetables, you will feel fuller, have more energy and think less about eating between meals. If you still feel the need for a little something to "hold you over" until your next meal, try a banana, an apple, or even a few grapes. You'll be amazed at the quick energy you get from these items.

10). Cereals, breads and rolls...

All of these items are excellent sources of nutrition and generally quite low in fat. The need to check their fat content does still exist, though. Some manufactures use large amounts of oil in their breads and cereals, thus significantly raising the fat content. Never assume that a product is low in fat just because the label says it is healthy for you. We are in dire need in this country for honesty in labeling food products. It is very easy to find breads and cereals with a fat content of only one or two grams per serving. These should be the only ones you regularly use.

Use this Page to list your favorite foods...

Use these tables located throughout this book to compile a useful list of items which currently account for your average daily fat intake (DFI).

Product Name	Quantity	Fat Grams

Using this list, check your cupboards and fridge to obtain the fat content of each of these items and write it down next to each line item for future reference.

(7)

OH NUTS!

Nuts:

Thus far I have avoided discussing the use of nuts as a part of your regular meals. This is due to the fact that it is very difficult to eat nuts and stay low fat. Ounce for ounce, nuts have one of the highest fat contents you can find. I have often joked with my wife about eating nuts as "taking Fat Pills". This may seem like a joke but the fact is, most nuts will exceed 225 grams of fat per pound. To put that in perspective, you would have to eat approximately 20 servings (3 ounces each) of your favorite steak to equal the fat content in one 8 ounce can of your favorite nuts My favorite peanut butter is 9 grams per tablespoon. This means that I can have a peanut butter and jelly sandwich, but it has to be considered the main meal of the day.

A single small handful of nuts will usually exceed 20 grams of fat, thus, I find it hard to recommend the regular use of nuts if you are trying to eat on a low fat budget.

Oils (Salad and Cooking)

Choose a vegetable oil which is low in saturated fat and high in polyunsaturated or monounsaturated fats. Fat, however, in either form, is still fat and the free use of any oils is not advisable. I would recommend that you calculate any oils that you use into your daily allowance of fat. It is important to note that many of the partially prepared foods you buy in the store are easy to convert to low-fat simply by eliminating the oil from the ingredients the recipe calls for and substituting 1% low-fat milk for the regular milk. Some people prefer to substitute applesauce for the oil. It sounds bizarre but it's actually not a bad alternative. Especially in cakes and muffins. Recently, I made a box of Potatoes Au Gratin that called for butter and milk. By substituting water and 1% low-fat milk for the butter called for in the recipe, I was able to reduce the fat content from 6 grams per serving down to just over 1 gram per serving.

The scenario just mentioned is not unusual. If you check the package of the food you are about to prepare, often there is nutritional information for the product in its present state and in its "as prepared" state. From this information it is easy to substitute and calculate the savings in grams of fat for each of the products servings. This chart below illustrates the difference in food values when these potatoes are prepared as directed. Notice the "fat" increase!

	Popular Potatoes Au Gratin Mix	Mix W/ Butter and Milk
Calories	90	140
Protein (g)	2	3
Fat (g)	1	6
Sodium (mg)	520	470
Potassium (mg)	210	170

From looking at this label, you can see that the fat is increased by 5 grams per serving when you add the milk and butter to the list of ingredients. Thus, by substituting low-fat or no-fat products in their place, you can reduce their fat content by as much as that same 5 grams. These numbers are from an actual label. When I made these potatoes, I used water in place of the butter and 1% milk in place of the regular milk, thereby increasing the fat content of the mix alone only very slightly (approximately 1 ½ grams for a total of only 1 ¼ grams of fat per serving). The beauty of it is, they still tasted great. I have found that oil generally adds very little to the taste of a product. Milk and butter add to the taste but if the product already has a strong flavor of its own, you won't notice much difference.

Cheese(s):

Herein lies my weakness. I love cheese – from cheese pizza right down to a "Baby Swiss" on some crackers. There's no denying it, I really love cheese. Unfortunately, I have thus far been unsuccessful in my search for a good low-fat cheese. In the battle of the bulging waistline, this was perhaps my most ominous foe! Knowing I will never defeat my desire for cheese, I conceded to form a truce. I agreed not to try to give cheese up entirely but I limit the use of it significantly in my daily eating. In return, I will allow myself a cheese "fantasy" without bonds periodically on a predetermined date and time. This way, I can still look forward to indulging without the negative side effects of eating it on a daily basis.

So far this method has been quite successful! I will typically indulge myself about twice a month and only eat one meal each time. This "fix" will usually sustain me for a couple of weeks. On a semi-daily basis, I have found a brand of cheese that contains only about 2 grams per one ounce slice. This is acceptable in sandwiches but on its own it is only fair at best.

Beverages:

Generally speaking, most beverages are fat-free. However, coffee, and tea (if they have milk or cream) can add significantly enough to your daily fat intake (DFI) to warrant monitoring. Little things add up very quickly! List the beverages you normally consume on a daily basis below.

Product Name	Quantity	Fat Grams

Use these tables located throughout this book to compile a useful list of items which currently account for your average daily fat intake (DFI).

OBSERVATIONS ON LOSING WEIGHT

One of the most important purchases you can make with regards to any weight loss or maintenance program is an accurate scale. My favorite is the sliding weight "doctor's variety". Although they are very expensive, it will be instrumental in determining your rate of weight loss and in calculating your daily nutritional needs. The test of a good scale is to get the same reading three or more times in a row. I have seen scales that will not only give three different readings for three tries but with fluctuations as great as 8 pounds. How anyone could take a weight program seriously while using such an inaccurate scale is truly beyond my comprehension.

When I first purchased my new scale, I tested it by weighing myself three times and then drinking a 4 ounce glass of water and repeated the process. The first three readings were the same and all three of the second readings confirmed the 4 ounce increase from the water. I thus concluded that this scale was sufficiently accurate. Purchasing this scale was instrumental in helping me to understand what was happening (or the "cause and effect") of my new eating style. It was because of this scale that I made some interesting discoveries.

It quickly became very apparent that I could not use the scale as a means to alter my weight. Or to put that another way, if I ate to please the scale, I would often find myself eating irregularly – too little at first, and later, too much. By checking my weight before and after each meal, before bedtime and when I first got up, I noticed a certain pattern developing.

Observation #1

If I failed to drink enough fluids the preceding day my weight loss would drop to as low as ½ a pound. Thus if I ate and drank to please the scale, I would sometimes deprive myself of the fluids my body obviously needed to digest properly and much to my dismay, the net result was often unfavorable.

Observation #2

While following this program, you will lose progressively less weight each day and then suddenly drop two to four pounds almost overnight. Don't get discouraged when you know you are eating wisely yet your weight loss seems to have stopped. Keep eating properly and before you know it, you'll drop almost into a different weight bracket on your scale.

Observation #3

Good nutrition needs to become a habit in order to be truly successful; therefore, you must regiment yourself to eating at regular times each day. Then, even if you are not really hungry, you should make yourself eat at meal times, as much food as you would typically eat. I believe many of us are deceived into believing that we are going to lose a "little weight" when we inadvertently skip a meal now and then. Nothing could be further from the truth, when we skip meals; the usual net effect is a gain in weight. This is due to an over-compensation factor. When we get overly hungry, our appetite becomes overly stimulated and requires much more food than normal to be satiated.

A good analogy to this would be improperly dressing for cold weather in the winter. Consider this scenario. Take a 20 minute walk outside on a cold winter day without adequate clothing. Although upon returning from your walk into the warmth of your home you may put on a sweater, (the same sweater that had you been wearing while walking would have kept you perfectly warm.) The amount of time necessary to feel warm again will far exceed the time it took you to achieve this level of discomfort. The human body is an incredibly resilient creation and it will not be slighted (not even by ourselves).

Considering how much of our lives was spent cultivating our misguided eating habits, it seems logical that the most effective way to get back on track again is by starting over. Thus, the title of this book..."Learning To Eat (Again)." The concept, to some, may seem a bit uncomfortable and perhaps even a little condescending. However, there is a good analogy to put this concept into perspective.

Our U.S. Constitution is revered by most Americans as an incredible document. It has survived for hundreds of years and is as true today as the day it was conceived. However, as times changed, amendments needed to be implemented to accommodate the new situations. Learning how to eat again is really the same scenario. Our parents and grandparents certainly didn't have access to the same level of prepared foods that we have today. As a result, there was no way they could pass down the information about this matter to their children and grandchildren.

The good news is, there is now a growing awareness that things need to change. The "Food Pyramid" has been declared obsolete and public access to information (now aided by the Internet) is growing faster than ever before. People WILL be learning to eat again!

Perhaps of all the eating habits that have changed over the past few generations, the availability of "snacks" is the most dramatic. With all of the new multi-billion dollar industries producing millionaires overnight while promoting new "fad" beverages and snacks, we need to be especially careful to learn about the content of these products. Which brings us to the next section about snacks. Use the space below to list all of the snacks you currently enjoy. Then try to locate the information about fat content and the appropriate amount which you typically consume. Refer back to this page to update as other ideas "come to mind".

Product Name	Quantity	Fat Grams

Use these tables located throughout this book to compile a useful list of items which currently account for your average daily fat intake (DFI).

(9)

SNACKING

Snacking is another way that we get ourselves into trouble. Snacks are permissible but should be done at the same time as we are eating the rest of our meal. In other words, as a dessert. If we want to incorporate a snack into our meal as a dessert, it will simply get digested along with the rest of our meal. However, when we eat inadvertently between meals, it throws off the body's normal cycle of digestion and thus promotes skipping meals. This ultimately results in gaining weight and improper nutrition.

Overweight people aren't overly- nourished, they are overweight as a result of poor eating habits and improper nutrition. The exception to this, of course, is the individual who is overweight due to a serious medical condition. I am speaking in the general sense and not as the only rule. The general attitude of a person viewed as being overweight is usually that of a person who eats really well. The fact of the matter is that if the person really ate well, he or she probably wouldn't be overweight. If however, when you first start to practice eating low-fat, you feel the strong need for a snack; try a piece of fruit or a glass of water. In addition, there are a lot of low fat snacks that you can implement into your daily routine as well. e.g. Fat free frozen yogurts and sorbets. Beware of the possible side effects of sodas and diet sodas. I have found that they can actually stimulate your appetite instead of satisfy it.

WEIGHT MAINTENANCE

Once you have achieved your ideal weight, you will need to adjust your eating habits to assure that you don't continue to lose weight. At this time, you may want to reintroduce some of the foods presently too high in fat, back into your diet. This time, however, on a more limited scale. Using this method, I hope you will find that you can control your weight so easily that you eventually don't even have to think about it. It will become second nature.

Unlike conventional dieting methods, monitoring your DFI does not require that you sometimes leave the table hungry. In addition, calorie monitoring becomes a "thing of the past". Because you can eat all the food your body needs to feel satisfied, maintaining your weight no longer needs to be a burden. This is why DFI monitoring will succeed where other methods have failed! Any method that forces you to deprive yourself continually will ultimately fail.

Reducing your daily fat intake is not at all the same as depriving yourself of the food your body needs. The fact is… in all likelihood, your body will receive more of the foods that it requires as a direct result of monitoring and limiting your DFI! Do not be surprised if you find yourself eating more fruits, grains and vegetables in an average day than you previously would have consumed in several days or perhaps even an entire week. To the best of my knowledge, there is no way that you can limit your daily fat intake to less than 20 grams per day and satisfy your body's appetite unless you increase your daily intake of fruits, grains and vegetables.

This process is actually enjoyable if you make a conscious effort to begin stocking your favorite fruits, grains and vegetables in various forms such as canned, dried, frozen, fresh or whatever. The objective is to avoid extra fat grams.

(11)

SETTING GOALS

Setting goals is a must. However, adjust your goals to work with your body's needs. The first week you may find that it is easy to lose as many as ten pounds. However, after the initial loss, the progress is usually much less dramatic. Resist the urge to starve yourself for the sake of losing additional weight; this will ultimately lead to disaster.

Instead, eat sufficiently at each meal so you can walk away completely satisfied. Not stuffed. But completely satisfied. Make your goals long-term and be flexible to accommodate your body's needs. You must first determine your own personal nutritional needs before you can make any demands on yourself to lose "X" number of pounds per week (or even per month).

Once you've established the rate of weight loss that is most desirable for you, it will be easier to set short-term goals. I would advise you to take the first week to document what you are eating on a regular basis currently. Once you have done this, you can accurately determine your daily fat intake (DFI). You can then develop a strategy which will allow you to reduce your DFI over a period of a few weeks to ultimately get down to the "20" grams level. I promise it will not be at all difficult if you proceed gradually. Lets say, for example, that you determine your current level of DFI to be 160 grams per day (DFI). If you reduce that level to 80 for week one and 40 for week two, by the beginning of week three, you will be at the optimal level of 20 grams DFI. Meanwhile, you will still be losing weight during the first two weeks as well.

IMPORTANT NOTE: *If your progress suddenly slows down, chances are, something has breached your "low fat radar". Carefully re-examine all of the consumed foods and eliminate any suspicious products.*

(12)

WATER

Several years ago, my father made a statement regarding the attitude of the general public towards prepackaged foods and beverages. He said "people will buy anything". In fact, if you put water in a can, they'd probably buy that too!" I think of this statement often now whenever I see a "bottled water" truck driving down the road. Bottled water has become a major part of our culture.

For some it is a necessity, for others a novelty and/or a convenience. In many instances, bottled water costs more than many of the popular soft drinks. Although I am not a bottled water customer at the time of this writing, there is very little question that society has gained a heightened awareness of the value of water for maintaining good health. As Nature's first "soft drink", it needs no improvement. It contains no artificial colors or sweeteners. It is lower in calories than any diet drink (0 calories) and it is totally fat free. Best of all, you can find it almost everywhere.

Water is absolutely essential to proper nutrition. It can be used as an appetite suppressant between meals. The free and liberal use of water will aid in your search for "good nutrition". Strive to replace your other beverages with water whenever possible. In addition to all the other benefits derived from drinking water liberally, it will help to "flush" your system of unwanted impurities. I find six to eight glasses per day to be my personal preference. Your need will likely vary and water contains no fat, therefore I will not recommend a specific amount to use.

(13)

CHEATING AND "DAYS OFF"

Provision should be made for days off or "cheating" as some people call it. A couple of times a month allow yourself that indulgence. However, do it at a regular meal time so as not to destroy your pattern of eating at appropriate times.

Should you choose to cheat for the entire day, be aware that your body may not like the splurge as much as your taste buds might lead you to believe. It is quite easy to make yourself sick from overindulgence, therefore, use good judgment. Foods which are rich in fat can be consumed so quickly that, if you aren't careful, you can eat a lot more than you had ever intended.

Holidays and parties or special occasions are good times to schedule your "cheating days" on. Keep in mind that you can enjoy yourself without totally losing your mind. I am telling you this out of personal conviction from past experiences. On more than one occasion, I went beyond the line of sanity and ate "all I wanted"! This was not a good idea! I realized very quickly that my body does not particularly like rich food as much as my taste buds would have me believe. Since then, I have learned that "cheating" within realistic boundaries you set for yourself makes much more sense. Setting realistic, predetermined, limits such as only one or two servings of cheesecake (as opposed to the whole cake) will allow you to enjoy the splurge without destroying your progress.

While eating high-fat foods, I have found that it is possible to gain weight at an incredibly fast rate. In some instances as much as four pounds in a single day! Your numbers may vary but it is amazing how fast it adds up!

Use this chart below to list the types of foods you will reserve for your "Cheating Days".

Product Name	Quantity	Fat Grams

Use these tables located throughout this book to compile a useful list of items which currently account for your average daily fat intake (DFI).

(14)

EATING OUT

With countless numbers of "fast food" chains professing good nutrition these days, it would seem that eating out could be easier than preparing your own healthy meals at home. Easier, perhaps but healthier is another story altogether.

Be forewarned, it is not easy to eat out *and* eat low-fat. If you are able to settle for a salad perhaps, but if you opt for any of the foods that traditionally made eating out so popular to begin with, you may have a problem. It is for this reason that I am recommending to you that you use one of the days off or "cheating days" when you do eat out. That way you don't have to concern yourself with counting fat grams.

To give credit where credit is due, "McDonald's" is one of the very few restaurants that have made a legitimate effort towards reducing fat from some of their main items. The menu does however still contain mostly high-fat foods and thus, caution is still advised. But if you are selective,it is possible to buy a reasonably healthy meal.

A good "rule of thumb" when eating out is to always choose a restaurant which lists nutritional information for each item on the menu someplace in the restaurant. If this information is unavailable, find another place to eat. Unfortunately, this may not be a small request. Very few establishments have "caught on" to consumer awareness of fat contents thus far. But take heart! There are more restaurants catching on all the time.

Beware of manufacturers of Donuts that are "baked fresh daily!" To the best of my knowledge, this is an outright lie! Donuts are almost always deep fried, (extremely high in fat) not baked. Baked donuts would be great! Please be sure to let me know if you ever find any.

(15)

SHOPPING FOR LOW-FAT FOODS

Fortunately, low-fat and no-fat foods are now quite abundant. There are cakes, pastries, cookies, crackers, ice cream, and puddings. You can also find several varieties of popcorn, breads, cheeses, pastas, sauces, hot dogs and T.V. Dinners. Basically, just about any food you can think of (and some that you might not have ever considered). Most of these are now available in either low or no-fat versions. The key is learning how to use them to fit into your new eating style.

When choosing a low-fat item, try to determine how the manufacturer reduced the fat. Did they eliminate the egg yolks or oil? Did they substitute skim milk for the whole milk? What about fat substitutes (such as Olestra, Caprenin, Salatrim or Sucrose Polyester) as well as other unnatural additives? Natural methods of reducing fat contents would obviously be preferred.

Always limit your use of products when you are unsure of the ingredients. You are, by far, better off eating foods that are as close as possible to their natural state. With fresh fruits, grains and vegetables at the top of your list, you should then proceed to complete your shopping list with healthy low-fat equivalents for all of your regular favorite foods.

WEEKLY MEAL PLANNER

SUNDAY

Breakfast_____

Lunch_____

Dinner_____

MONDAY

Breakfast_____

Lunch_____

Dinner_____

TUESDAY

Breakfast_____

Lunch_____

Dinner_____

WEDNESDAY

Breakfast_____

Lunch_____

Dinner_____

THURSDAY

Breakfast_____

Lunch_____

Dinner_____

FRIDAY

Breakfast_____

Lunch_____

Dinner_____

SATURDAY (FREE DAY)

SHOPPING LIST

FRUIT...

_____Apples _____ Bananas _____Melons _____Oranges

_____Peaches _____Pears _____Pineapple ___Grapes

_____Plums _____Nectarines ___Cherries ___Tangerines

Other _____

VEGETABLES...

_____Lettuce _____Tomatoes _____Cucumbers

_____Broccoli _____Cauliflower _____ Radishes

_____Celery ____Bell Peppers____Green Beans____Squash

_____Wax Beans _____Eggplant _____Onions _____Peas

_____Brussel Sprouts _____Asparagus _____Mushrooms

_____Carrots _____ Potatoes _____Other

GRAINS...

Cereal type _____ _____

_____ _____

Bread_____   Rolls_____ Muffins_____

Crackers_____   Flour_____Pastry _____

Pasta_____   Rice _____

Other _____

MISCELLANEOUS...

Dairy products_____

Meat products _____

Desserts_____

Beverages_____

Baking needs_____

Household supplies _____

Other _____

Note; Always prepare a shopping list in advance based on your current
inventory and your "Weekly meal planner".

WEEKLY MEAL PLANNER (*Sample*)

SUNDAY

Breakfast.... Cereal w/ 1% milk, 1 apple, toast
w/jam .... Fat 4 Grams

Lunch... Spaghetti w/ sauce, 3 oz. chicken, green
beans.. Fat 8 Grams

Dinner... Salad, mashed potatoes w/ gravy, 3
vegetables..…...... Fat 1 Grams

MONDAY

Breakfast... Fruit salad, 1 bagel, 6 oz. orange
juice... Fat 3 Grams

Lunch... Vegetable Pizza, bowl of soup…................... Fat 6 Grams

Dinner... Tuna & Potato salad, Lettuce & tomato sandwich.....
………..…...…… Fat 6 Grams

TUESDAY

Breakfast... Non-fat pancakes w/fruit…...................... Fat 0 Grams

Lunch... English muffin pizzas, vegetable
soup……….. Fat 8 Grams

Dinner... Pasta salad, turkey sandwich ……….............. Fat 7 Grams

WEDNESDAY

Breakfast... French toast, 8 oz. 1% milk...................... Fat 8 Grams

Lunch... Tomato soup, low-fat rolls............................ Fat 4 Grams

Dinner... Chicken fajitas...… Fat 8 Grams

THURSDAY

Breakfast... Oatmeal w/ raisins, 2 low-fat
muffins... Fat 5 Grams

Lunch... 2 sandwiches w/ lettuce/ tomato/ low-fat
meat... Fat 10 Grams

Dinner... Beans & Corn succotash, green & wax beans..
....…… Fat 2 Grams

FRIDAY

Breakfast... 1 pouched egg on toast, orange juice..... Fat 10 Grams

Lunch... American chop suey, French bread,
salad... Fat 8 Grams

Dinner... Fresh fruit, low-fat cottage cheese............... Fat 2 Grams

SATURDAY (FREE DAY)

Note: I use the Monday menu to revolve the weekly schedule.

Preparation Instructions

In the pages that follow, I will explain how to prepare the meals in a manner that is consistent with the allocations of "Fat" grams on the preceding pages. *It is not my intention to give specific recipes* but rather to demonstrate various methods for controlling fat contents in your daily food preparation.

Sunday

Breakfast... Cereal w/ 1% milk, 1 apple, toast w/jam

Many breakfast cereals contain only one or two grams of fat per serving. Half of one cup of 1% low-fat milk contains only one gram of fat. Choose a bread that contains only one gram of fat (or less) per slice and substitute jelly or jam in place of the butter or margarine. Enjoy as many apples as you would like.

Lunch... Spaghetti w/ sauce, 3 oz. chicken, green beans

For lunch, prepare your spaghetti (Regular or "no-yolk") without any oil and choose a low-fat or no-fat sauce. Grill, bake, broil or stew approximately 3 oz. of fresh chicken breast with the skin removed. Enjoy all the green beans (or similar vegetable) that you desire.

Dinner... Salad, mashed potatoes w/ gravy, 3 vegetables

For dinner, try a multi-vegetable salad with non-fat salad dressing. Experiment with various brands to find the type which best suits your taste. The mashed potatoes should be prepared with 1% low-fat milk (or skim milk if you prefer) and topped with low-fat gravy. There are many types available which contain only one gram or less per serving. Accompany the potatoes and gravy with an assortment of three of your favorite vegetables. Do not limit yourself to only one or two favorite vegetables. You can use their color as a guide to get the best nutritional balance.

Monday

Breakfast… Fruit salad, 1 bagel, 6 oz. orange juice

For breakfast, try a freshly made fruit salad using melon balls, citrus sections, apples, grapes, cherries, bananas and any other favorite fruits. Be creative. Try warming your bagel in the toaster by adjusting your toaster to a "lighter setting" and enjoy your bagel with your fruit without the need for butter, margarine or cream cheese. Choose a fruit Juice that will go well with your salad.

Lunch… Vegetable Pizza, bowl of soup

Many stores carry ready-made pizza dough. Using one of these, try topping it with tomato sauce and your favorite vegetables. This type of pizza is extremely quick and easy to prepare. For your soup, choose a soup that is only one or two grams of fat. The number of slices of pizza you have will be determined by the fat content in your soup. Typically, homemade vegetable pizza will contain one to three grams per slice. Determine the fat content in your creation by adding the total grams of fat in each ingredient you are using and then divide by the number of slices you are cutting the pie into. Remember, if the fat content is higher than you expected, you can always divide the pizza into smaller slices.

Dinner... Tuna and Potato salad, Lettuce & tomato sandwich.

Fat contents for tuna packed in water are dramatically lower than tuna which is packed in oil. When preparing your salad, always use tuna packed in water and fat-free salad dressing or mayonnaise. Next, peel and boil a few potatoes, chop up some onions and parsley if you'd like and combine the ingredients with the fat-free mayonnaise and tuna for a great tasting salad which you can indulge in as much as you'd like. Each serving typically contains only one gram of fat (compare this to regular tuna potato salad which can contain as much as 40 grams per serving). Using a hearty low-fat bread, spread non-fat mayonnaise or salad dressing on the bread in place of butter or margarine. Then simply slice up some fresh beef-steak tomatoes and your favorite lettuce for a refreshing sandwich which is healthy and satisfying.

Tuesday

Breakfast... Non-fat pancakes w/fruit

You may ask "how can you possibly make pancakes without any fat in them"? I had wondered the same thing. A few months ago, I decided to experiment to see if I could find a way to make pancakes that were low in fat. The first step was to eliminate the oil that most favorite recipes call for and see what would happen. Surprisingly, the lack of oil was determined to be barely perceptible. The next problem was figuring out a way to cook them without any oils. I was pleased to discover that with reasonable care and a high quality non-stick frying pan, this feat is in fact possible. Timing, however, is everything. Be careful not to try flipping them too soon or you may mangle them. By experimenting as to the time needed to turn them over without disaster, I acquired a "feel" for cooking them with few casualties. Generally speaking, most pancake syrups contain no fat. If your have no particular concern about sugar consumption, enjoy all of these pancakes that you would like. If sugar is a concern, consider using a fruit compote or your favorite brand of "spreadable" fruit.

Lunch... English muffin pizzas, vegetable soup

Pizza made using English muffins is one of the easiest meals you can prepare. Simply split the muffins into halves and spread some tomato sauce on each half and sprinkle small portions of your favorite toppings on. Use any toppings you normally would but remember to monitor the fat content of each "pizza". The total fat should not exceed 8 grams. Be aware that English muffins have some fat also. Thus, if you want only one piece of pizza, use all 8 grams. For two pieces they must not exceed 4 grams each and so on...you are on an honor system here, please don't cheat yourself.

If you can't prepare a particular meal without exceeding your allowable fat level, you can always exceed the limit and compensate later the same day by reducing your limit on another item. The key here is moderation. You may desire to use a topping such as mozzarella cheese. By adding a sprinkling only, you could limit the additional fat increase to as little as 1 additional gram. However, if you allow your taste buds to overrule your sense of reason, you could easily increase the override by 20 grams or more! When faced with this kind of dilemma, consider that you can eat more units without gaining more fat if you use moderation.

e.g. Consider this; you just prepared two pizzas containing three grams of fat each before adding cheese. By adding only a light sprinkling of cheese to each one you will increase the fat content by approximately 1 gram each to give you a grand total of eight grams for both. This amount still fits into your daily allowance with perhaps only a minor adjustment needed if you are still having soup with that meal. However, should you choose to heap the cheese on "Pizzeria" style, you could be increasing the fat to over 20 grams per serving. There is no possible way that you can make an adjustment for that much excess. Your only alternatives would be to eat one-half of one English muffin pizza for approximately 12 grams of fat and walk away from the meal hungry, or to declare a "cheat" day. If you have been diligent for the preceding week or two you may seriously consider the latter.

If you find yourself declaring more than two or three "cheat days" per month, you should consider making an adjustment to your DFI it could be that you are reducing your level at too rapid a pace. It would be better to readjust your intake to a higher daily level than to continually "cheat" or even worse, abandon the monitoring altogether. The longer you monitor your DFI, the easier it becomes to regulate your intake. Having said that, consider a low-fat vegetable soup to accompany your pizzas. They can be found with less than one gram of fat per serving if desired.

Dinner... Pasta salad, turkey sandwich

Many people avoid pasta because they believe it is very fattening. The truth is, pasta is generally very low in fat, with typically only one to three grams of fat per serving. Depending upon the size of your appetite, you can find a pasta that works best for you. If you have a large appetite, like I do, you are better off purchasing a low fat variety so you can have more than one serving. If one serving is all you generally desire, almost any brand will suffice. I have no specific recipe for pasta salad. I will usually purchase a "dry mix" in the local store and prepare it without the additional oil they will usually call for. It is not difficult to find brands that will contain less than 2 grams per serving if you eliminate the high fat ingredients they advise you to add. A turkey sandwich is an excellent accompaniment to your pasta salad. By adding low-fat bread, fat free mayonnaise, fresh lettuce and tomatoes to "reduced fat" turkey slices, a delicious turkey sandwich will only add about 3 grams of fat to your meal.

Wednesday

Breakfast… French toast, 8 oz. 1% milk

By substituting a cholesterol free egg replacement in your favorite French toast recipe and using a non-stick cooking spray instead of oil, butter or margarine, you may not even feel like you are eating on a low-fat budget. Including an 8 oz. glass of milk with this meal (1% low-fat) you should find it possible to enjoy as many slices of French toast as you would like and still stay within your designated guidelines.

Lunch… Tomato soup, low-fat rolls

Tomato soup is usually low-fat or no-fat. Please resist the urge to use butter on your low-fat rolls. Butter and margarine are almost pure fat. If you remind yourself of this fact each time you reach for the butter knife, you will do well.

Dinner… Chicken fajitas

Steam two flour tortillas (be sure to watch the fat contents when purchasing, they can run as high as 4 grams of fat each). Then carefully fold in the following prepared ingredients.

Filling Ingredients (for the chicken fajitas)

Stir fry 6 oz. of chicken, some mushrooms, green and red bell peppers and onions using a non-stick pan and low-fat cooking spray or a light touch of oil (1-2 teaspoons) until chicken is fully cooked and tender. Divide into two equal portions and place ingredients on the center of each steamed tortilla. Fold carefully to allow fajitas to be held while eating.

Thursday

Breakfast… Oatmeal w/ raisins and 2 low-fat muffins

These items are almost self explanatory except for a brief reminder once again about using low-fat milk (on the oatmeal) and make sure to use the butter or margarine very sparingly if you prefer your muffins that way.

Lunch… 2 sandwiches w/ lettuce/ tomato/ low-fat meat

Substituting fat free mayonnaise or salad dressing for the butter or margarine you would normally use on your bread, generously laden your sandwiches with lettuce and tomatoes and then finish them off with one or two low-fat turkey slices. Fat percentages in both the turkey slices and the bread will vary. Choose brands that are only one or two grams of fat for each serving.

Dinner... Beans & Corn succotash, green & wax beans

All of these items are low in fat so you do not need to be concerned about the number of servings you consume. Whenever any scheduled meal calls strictly for vegetables, feel free to enjoy as much as you desire.

Friday

Breakfast... 1 Pouched Egg on toast, orange juice

A typical poached egg has 5 grams of fat. In this meal, I have made an allowance for using low-fat margarine on the toast. If you are content to have your toast without butter or margarine, you can have two servings instead of only one.

Lunch...American Chop Suey, French Bread and Salad

By making your own meals, you can dramatically influence the fat content in almost anything. In this example, if you use a low-fat pasta and a tomato sauce with "no" fat, by adding no additional fats or oils and adding a small portion of lean ground beef (well drained), you can easily keep the fat content within acceptable limits. The ground beef is used to flavor the meal just as you would normally use a seasoning. Remember to use a low fat or no fat salad dressing on your salad and eat the French bread with the American Chop Suey. If you use the tomato sauce like a dip, you can eliminate the need for butter or margarine.

Dinner...Fresh fruit, low-fat cottage cheese

Cottage cheese is presently available in very low fat varieties. You should have no problem finding a brand that contains only one or two grams of fat per serving.

With a little bit of creativity, virtually any meal can be prepared with the fat content dramatically reduced. The key to success is more about awareness and really doesn't require a particularly high level of skill.

Once you've seen the dramatic results which lowering fat contents will yield, you will likely be motivated to create many of your favorite meals in a "leaner" version.

The food manufacturers have produced many frozen meals that claim to be low in fat. Some of them are actually pretty decent. However, their idea of "low-fat" is still a bit on the high side in the overall scheme of the daily meal planning. Most of the more desirable meals contain over 10 grams of fat and the serving size is a bit skimpy for my needs. However, you may want to consider using one of these meals on occasion to give yourself a little break from cooking without needing to feel guilty about trashing your DFI level.

I would highly recommend that you consider stocking as many non-fat snack products in your home as soon as possible. This is especially important during the first few weeks of this program. There are many very desirable items available to choose from these days. If you can, make a special shopping trip to search for the products you know you would like to have available. Remember, Non-fat, not "low fat" snacks. That way you can have as many as you'd like at any given time.

(17)

CONCLUSION

In conclusion, regulating your daily fat intake (DFI) will make controlling your weight possible without the need for conventional dieting plans. Following the "common sense" guidelines set forth in the preceding chapters, it is easy to determine your own DFI needs.

You can now take a moment to review your charts listed earlier in the chapters. There are additional copies of the basic forms in the back of this book. Once you understand your own personal requirements, it becomes much easier to regulate your intake. Remember to start out by reducing your DFI by only 20% for the first week. Ultimately, the goal is to reduce your level of DFI to only 20 grams per day.

Dishonest labeling of many food items as well as false advertising by "fast food" chains has been instrumental in keeping us ignorant on this subject in the past. However, the future promises to be much brighter, now that we know the truth about fat contents in our food. With practice, anyone can easily learn to control their daily fat intake (DFI).

They say every great journey begins with a single step. You've already taken some important steps by looking for a solution, buying this book and reading it. You are now well on your way to lowering your DFI and taking control of your weight. You can do this. Good luck!

Please feel free to forward questions or comments to me at...

Feedback@brianvmenard.com

(18)

The following pages contain 4 weeks worth of meal planner pages which can be torn out and copied or used in the book.

(Tear out sheets for "weekly meal planner")
Located on the following pages.

(Tear out sheets for "weekly meal planner")
Located on the following pages.

(18)

WEEKLY MEAL PLANNER

SUNDAY

Breakfast_____

Lunch_____

Dinner_____

MONDAY

Breakfast_____

Lunch_____

Dinner_____

TUESDAY

Breakfast_____

Lunch_____

Dinner_____

(Tear out sheets for "weekly meal planner")
Located on the following pages.

WEDNESDAY

Breakfast_____

Lunch_____

Dinner_____

THURSDAY

Breakfast_____

Lunch_____

Dinner_____

FRIDAY

Breakfast_____

Lunch_____

Dinner_____

SATURDAY (FREE DAY)

(Tear out sheets for "weekly meal planner")
Located on the following pages.

WEEKLY MEAL PLANNER

SUNDAY

Breakfast_____

Lunch_____

Dinner_____

MONDAY

Breakfast_____

Lunch_____

Dinner_____

TUESDAY

Breakfast_____

Lunch_____

Dinner_____

(Tear out sheets for "weekly meal planner")
Located on the following pages.

WEDNESDAY

Breakfast_____

Lunch_____

Dinner_____

THURSDAY

Breakfast_____

Lunch_____

Dinner_____

FRIDAY

Breakfast_____

Lunch_____

Dinner_____

SATURDAY (FREE DAY)

(Tear out sheets for "weekly meal planner")
Located on the following pages.

WEEKLY MEAL PLANNER

SUNDAY

Breakfast_____

Lunch_____

Dinner_____

MONDAY

Breakfast_____

Lunch_____

Dinner_____

TUESDAY

Breakfast_____

Lunch_____

Dinner_____

(Tear out sheets for "weekly meal planner")
Located on the following pages.

WEDNESDAY

Breakfast_____

Lunch_____

Dinner_____

THURSDAY

Breakfast_____

Lunch_____

Dinner_____

FRIDAY

Breakfast_____

Lunch_____

Dinner_____

SATURDAY (FREE DAY)

(Tear out sheets for "weekly meal planner")
Located on the following pages.

WEEKLY MEAL PLANNER

SUNDAY

Breakfast_____

Lunch_____

Dinner_____

MONDAY

Breakfast_____

Lunch_____

Dinner_____

TUESDAY

Breakfast_____

Lunch_____

Dinner_____

(Tear out sheets for "weekly meal planner")
Located on the following pages.

WEDNESDAY

Breakfast_____

Lunch_____

Dinner_____

THURSDAY

Breakfast_____

Lunch_____

Dinner_____

FRIDAY

Breakfast_____

Lunch_____

Dinner_____

SATURDAY (FREE DAY)

The following pages can be "torn out"
for your weekly shopping list.

SHOPPING LIST

FRUIT…

_____Apples _____ Bananas _____Melons _____Oranges

_____Peaches _____Pears _____Pineapple ___Grapes

_____Plums _____Nectarines ___Cherries ___Tangerines

Other _____

VEGETABLES…

_____Lettuce _____Tomatoes _____Cucumbers

_____Broccoli _____Cauliflower _____Radishes

_____Celery _____Bell Peppers_____Green Beans_____Squash

_____Wax Beans _____Eggplant _____Onions _____Peas

_____Brussel Sprouts _____Asparagus _____Mushrooms

_____Carrots _____ Potatoes _____Other

GRAINS…

Cereal type _____ _____

_____ _____

Bread_____   Rolls_____ Muffins_____

Crackers_____   Flour_____Pastry _____

Pasta_____   Rice _____

Other _____

MISCELLANEOUS...

Dairy products_____

Meat products _____

Desserts_____

Beverages_____

Baking needs_____

Household supplies _____

Other _____

Note; Always prepare a shopping list in advance based on your current
inventory and your "Weekly meal planner".

SHOPPING LIST

FRUIT...

_____Apples _____ Bananas _____Melons _____Oranges

_____Peaches _____Pears _____Pineapple ___Grapes

_____Plums _____Nectarines ___Cherries ___Tangerines

Other _____

VEGETABLES...

_____Lettuce _____Tomatoes _____Cucumbers

_____Broccoli _____Cauliflower _____ Radishes

_____Celery ____Bell Peppers____Green Beans____Squash

_____Wax Beans _____Eggplant _____Onions _____Peas

_____Brussel Sprouts _____Asparagus _____Mushrooms

_____Carrots _____ Potatoes _____Other

GRAINS...

Cereal type _____ _____

_____ _____

Bread_____ Rolls_____ Muffins_____

Crackers_____ Flour_____Pastry _____

Pasta_____ Rice _____

Other _____

MISCELLANEOUS...

Dairy products_____

Meat products _____

Desserts_____

Beverages_____

Baking needs_____

Household supplies _____

Other _____

Note; Always prepare a shopping list in advance based on your current
inventory and your "Weekly meal planner".

SHOPPING LIST

FRUIT…

____Apples _____ Bananas _____Melons _____Oranges

____Peaches _____Pears _____Pineapple ___Grapes

____Plums _____Nectarines ___Cherries ___Tangerines

Other _____

VEGETABLES…

_____Lettuce _____Tomatoes _____Cucumbers

_____Broccoli _____Cauliflower _____ Radishes

_____Celery ____Bell Peppers____Green Beans____Squash

_____Wax Beans _____Eggplant _____Onions _____Peas

_____Brussel Sprouts _____Asparagus _____Mushrooms

_____Carrots _____ Potatoes _____Other

GRAINS…

Cereal type _____ _____

_____ _____

Bread_____   Rolls_____ Muffins_____

Crackers_____   Flour_____Pastry _____

Pasta_____   Rice _____

Other _____

MISCELLANEOUS...

Dairy products_____

Meat products _____

Desserts_____

Beverages_____

Baking needs_____

Household supplies _____

Other _____

Note; Always prepare a shopping list in advance based on
your current inventory and your "Weekly meal planner".

SHOPPING LIST

FRUIT...

____Apples _____ Bananas _____Melons _____Oranges

____Peaches _____Pears _____Pineapple ___Grapes

____Plums _____Nectarines ___Cherries ___Tangerines

Other _____

VEGETABLES...

_____Lettuce _____Tomatoes _____Cucumbers

_____Broccoli _____Cauliflower _____ Radishes

_____Celery ____Bell Peppers ____Green Beans____Squash

_____Wax Beans _____Eggplant _____Onions _____Peas

_____Brussel Sprouts _____Asparagus _____Mushrooms

_____Carrots _____ Potatoes _____Other

GRAINS...

Cereal type _____ _____

_____ _____

Bread_____ Rolls_____ Muffins_____

Crackers_____ Flour_____Pastry _____

Pasta_____ Rice _____

Other _____

MISCELLANEOUS...

Dairy products_____

Meat products _____

Desserts_____

Beverages_____

Baking needs_____

Household supplies _____

Other _____

Note; Always prepare a shopping list in advance based on
your current inventory and your "Weekly meal planner".

(20)

New Favorite Foods

Product Name	Quantity	Fat Grams

Use these tables to compile a useful list of items which currently account for your average daily fat intake (DFI).

New Favorite Foods

Product Name	Quantity	Fat Grams

Use these tables to compile a useful list of items which currently account for your average daily fat intake (DFI).

New Favorite Foods

Product Name	Quantity	Fat Grams

Use these tables to compile a useful list of items which currently account for your average daily fat intake (DFI).

New Favorite Foods

Product Name	Quantity	Fat Grams

Use these tables to compile a useful list of items which currently account for your average daily fat intake (DFI).

New Favorite Foods

Product Name	Quantity	Fat Grams

Use these tables to compile a useful list of items which currently account for your average daily fat intake (DFI).

New Favorite Foods

Product Name	Quantity	Fat Grams

Use these tables to compile a useful list of items which currently account for your average daily fat intake (DFI).

"Learning How To Eat (Again)"

Please feel free to forward questions or comments to me at...

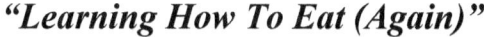

Feedback@brianvmenard.com